Praise for Kathleen's Work

I have received more helpful information from Kathleen Pagnini's class on the pelvic floor than I did from *all* the medical providers (Internists, OBGYNs, Urogynecologists) in the last 4 years!" — *Sherri, 80, Author, Actress*

After injuring my shoulders from over-exercising, I needed a new program that supported women over 60. I stopped those crazy workouts, and lost 20lbs. with Kathleen's program. — *Marcie, Japanese Acupressure Therapist, Scripps Hospitals, San Diego*

As a retired nurse practitioner with an OBGYN, I really understood the science, but never would have dreamed that such an easy method would have such phenomenal results. I was taking Vicodin for back pain twice a day for a year and feeling depressed. I am only 73 and was feeling 93! My Osteopath doctor introduced me to Kathleen. After the first two weeks of taking Kathleen's class, I didn't have to take Vicodin and I am not depressed anymore! Thanks to Kathleen I'm in it for the long term and couldn't be more thrilled! — *Linda, retired nurse practitioner*

I found Kathleen after I had my third child and my belly was sticking way out, (diastisis). I was in significant pain and my doctor said I would need surgery. Then I found kathleen and did private sessions with her for a few months. My belly is no longer huge and I have no more pain! — *Laura, mom of 3*

I found Kathleen and have been doing her classes and workshops and I must say that besides no more accidental leaking... my husband surely notices a difference with me sexually and loves this program too! — *Donna, Entrepreneur*

By age 48, I was having increased incontinence (despite never having children). My hip has arthritis and a cartilage tear and I have an unstable vertebra in my low back which was making walking painful. After my inner unit shut down almost 5 years ago I learned to function again using my large, powerful muscles which worked...sort of. I was holding myself so tightly to keep things together that I was continually inhibiting my deep core and exhausting myself.

Reversing that pattern has been huge! I can stand, walk and bend with much more safety/confidence and my incontinence is gone.

I cannot adequately express the positive impact this work has had on my body and my long term prognosis. I have benefitted tremendously by working with Kathleen. — *Kelly, Physical Therapist*

I haven't worn a two piece bathing suit since my son was born. I just didn't like the way my tummy looked after childbirth. Now, for the first time in 15 years, after working with Kathleen a short time, I am now able to wear a bikini...and I'm 50!" — *Bernadette, Bank Executive*

I have to tell you how much I have appreciated working with you, Kathleen. The things you have taught me I have put into practice with such success — personally and with patients. I thank the Lord for you and how He has used you to help me and my patients. — *Lynn, Physical Therapist*

After 20 sessions, I feel hopeful and more whole. A botched hysterectomy, endometriosis, a displaced hip joint, and an AS disease diagnosis left me pretty depressed. Kathleen has helped me find my inner strength physically, but the by-product is that I am stronger emotionally, as well. I keep the core of my life, family, priorities, and body much better in balance. Mind, Body and Spirit alignment is not what I thought I was purchasing, but in the end, it is what I have received. — *Carrie, grade school teacher*

7 Secrets to a *Sexy Silhouette*

Kathleen Pagnini

The Corset and The Coat
Redondo Beach, California

7 Secrets to a Sexy Silhouette

by Kathleen Pagnini

First published 2017

ISBN: 978-0-692-04458-2

Kathleen Pagnini

Email: kathleen@kathleenpagnini.com

Phone: 310-303-2714

www.TheCorsetandTheCoat.com

Original Illustrations Copyright © Kathleen Pagnini

Based on the work of Dr. Theresa Nesbitt, OB/GYN and is used with permission.

PHOTO CREDITS:

Cover Photo: Brian Ribbey

Author Photo, page 13: Jym Duane

The Corset and The Coat

Redondo Beach, Californina

Contents

Disclaimer

All information presented in this book is what I have learned from private mentorship with Dr. Theresa Nesbitt since 2009, and represents my current understanding of this revolutionary and science-based system. I am still on my journey in my efforts to refine yours.

Since the brain is always changing, read this book over and over to expedite your results, sign up for the 6 week online program at thecorsetandthecoat.com and devour Dr. Theresa Nesbitt's book, *Evolutionary Eating*.

This book gives general information on health and wellness and is not a substitute for health advice and medical care from your primary care physician and other medical professionals familiar with your specific history and circumstances. Please seek such specific health and medical advice before making significant changes in your diet, daily routine or fitness activities, especially if you are under a physician's care for other medical conditions.

Suggested Books for Additional Reading

> The Brain that Changes Itself, Norman Doidge
>
> Deep Nutrition, Catherine Shanahan
>
> Move a Little Lose a Lot, James Levine

For more info on scientific-based research, please email the author at: kathleen@kathleenpagnini.com

Acknowledgments

I AM VERY VERY GRATEFUL for all of the hours and years Dr. Theresa Nesbitt OB/GYN, has devoted to privately mentoring me on women's wellness: how to stop the leaks, back pain, sexual dysfunction and belly fat without pills, pads, surgery, Kegels or crunches. This work has not only changed my life on so many levels but also the lives of my clients. My confidence and self-respect has increased exponentially as I learn more about this under-worked and under-appreciated part of our anatomy that we didn't even know existed. There were dauntless days and nights she spent teaching me what I needed to understand to be able to help other women. My deepest appreciation and respect goes out to this woman, my friend, and business partner of many talents! I am grateful far beyond words can express.

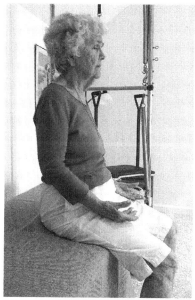

My mom doing the Reed exercise.

I am also very thankful to have been blessed with a wonderful mother, Camille Zvonek Pagnini, May She Rest In Peace. A writer, poet, artist, and lover of babies (I am one of eight), she had endless curiosity in everything. She taught me the value of seeking joy in all and to always look for the good in people. This advice has helped me immensely throughout my worldly travels. But most of all, she taught me to stay faithful, trust God, laugh often, and to always have fun and be goofy. Thank you dear mum! This book is for you!

Valuable Bonuses Just for Buyers of

7 Secrets to a Sexy Silhouette

Helping you get your body in shape — at any age — is my driving passion and that's why, as a reader of this book, I want you to experience first-hand what's possible for you.

MY GIFT TO YOU:

2 Free Videos to Get You Started on Your Path to a Sexy Silhouette

Video 1:
A Tour of Your Pelvis and Your Pelvic Floor

This video will take you through the basics of understanding your "Inner Corset". You must understand this part of your anatomy and why it's so vital to your health.

Video 2:
How to sit at your desk for less peeing, pain and pooch while balancing hormones for less belly fat and droopy body parts.

No pills, pads, surgery, kegels or crunches required!

Claim Your Bonus Videos at
KathleenPagnini.com/book-bonus

Introduction

> *"Be faithful in small things for it is in them that your strength lies."*
>
> *Mother Teresa*

*I*t took me over 35 years as an international Fitness and Pilates expert to discover that I was doing things backwards. I was forcing a shape from the outside and telling my clients to do the same when it's exactly the opposite!

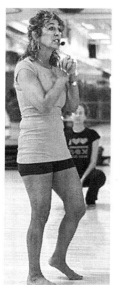

I have been training only half of the core, the outer core muscles, all these years for a shape, without a clue of another whole core inside, which was responsible for my shape and has always been there. I just didn't know it and have been patching a tire without even knowledge of an inner tube, over and over again.

And worse, I was telling people to do the same. "Squeeze this, engage that," without a clue I was making things worse for them long term, like back pain, increased leaking, more belly bulge and so much more that I had to stop!

I am not a physical therapist or a doctor, just a curious 35-year fitness and Pilates expert whose curiosity made the best of her, and was invited to mentor privately with the developer/inventor of this program to show the women of the world this priceless treasure that already exists inside.

It's not easy being a pioneer, but the benefits are way too fast and amazing that I have to share this sooner than later!

I've already done the hard part and have blazed a shortcut for you!

It was a Saturday morning in September when I rushed in late to what was going to be the most pivotal and life-changing workshop in my life.

It was 2009. I had just finished creating a DVD called Pilates and Chocolate and 5 Secrets to a Sexier You, and was ready to go after my next dream, which was to live by the beach and be a core trainer for the Chicago Bulls.

I moved to San Diego and right away was urged by my Pilates mentor in Scottsdale, to go to a workshop in San Diego given by Dr. Theresa Nesbitt, OB/GYN Women's Wellness Specialist, Chicago based.

The information she presented I had never heard before, yet had me intrigued from the moment she spoke. She spoke of another core, an inner core, and showed a video of a baby with diapers holding on to a table while dancing (mirroring – mimicking) Beyoncé's dance moves to "Single Ladies." I had no clue why she was showing this video and what it had to do with this inner core she was talking about. Regardless, I sat there mesmerized by the plethora of information!

The weekend workshop ended and I went up to Dr. Theresa, graciously thanked her, and gave her a copy of my Pilates DVD.

A month passed and I got THE CALL! Yes, the Chicago Bulls wanted to interview me to be a core trainer! I was so excited. I emailed Dr. Theresa and asked if she could possibly help me with the interview, since it was her town.

She invited me to come to Chicago to help me with the interview. She mentioned her dad owned the Memphis Grizzlies so I thought, "How serendipitous! This is even better than I thought!"

It was winter when I went to Chicago. Dr. Theresa and I hiked through the snow on her property talking core.

The first thing she said is "First of all, Kathleen, athletes don't even train their true core, they are training only the wrapping. The outside."

At that point, I was completely lost! I thought I knew everything about the core. I got great results with my Pilates clients, they kept coming back for more... and now she's telling me there's another core and it included the pelvic floor muscles? I had to know more!

She said, "You have another whole core and you can't train it like a sit up or bicep curl. It's trained better with imagery and intention!"

What?! I just spent $10,000 of hard Pilates earned cash to create a DVD about the core!

So what was this? There was more to the core? A whole other one? Imagery and intention? What?

I realized I DID know everything about the core, *half* of it that is.

During the weekend, Dr. Theresa said that in 20 years there was going to be an epidemic of incontinence, and baby boomers would be going into nursing homes for leaking urine only, they can't make it to the bathroom and the doctor codes it mobility issues. The fact is age doesn't have anything to do with holding the pee. We should always be able to MAKE it to the loo. She added that we are also doing things with our bodies that are making this problem worse and we have been for years! She asked if I would be interested in helping her pioneer this revolutionary science-based 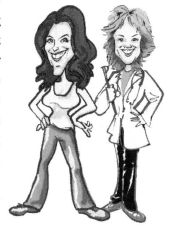 program for women to help them with the leaks, back pain, and increased sexuality, WITHOUT PILLS PADS SURGERY OR KEGELS. I thought about it for a half a second and said, "YES! I will help!"

The rest is history.

I never did go to the interview. There was another whole core I needed to learn about, and then I had to teach the ladies first!

"They call it the change of life, the fact is it's about what you look like, what you feel like and never losing your independence. To be a person of value and worth, it's what being a woman is all about."

Dr. Theresa Nesbitt, OBGYN/Women's Wellness Specialist

In order to have a new look, we must look where we haven't looked before.

It's not that what you have been doing is wrong: it's all perspective; we are always trying to improve.

If you are my age, in your 50s and beyond and tired of the workouts not working, the Kegels not holding back your pee, the annoying pain that's getting worse and increasing sexual difficulties and want to avoid a future of pills, pads, surgery, more pointless workouts or prescribed Kegels.

THIS BOOK IS FOR YOU!

On the other hand, if you're my age, in your 50s and beyond, love spending hours in the gym or working out and the results it yields, feeling and functioning like you're a 20-year old already, then this book is NOT for you.

For this, I feel blessed and honored beyond words to be a part of this new revolution for women's health and shape, without all the crazy diets, pills, pads, surgery, cardio, or crunches. It's just the way we work, plain and simple. You can learn now or later, you choose, but this revolutionary science-based program already in Europe has arrived.

Dr. Theresa calls the inner core the Corset, and the outer core the Coat.

The problem is that the inner core, Corset, has become loose and fails to tighten properly. It helps you hold your posture and organize your body, keeping things in and up so everything is in its place.

But, you have been duct taping your body together for many years, using only the outside muscles to hold and organize your body, until you reboot and reclaim your bounce, youth and vitality, your Corset.

The Chicago Bulls job was a great opportunity, but they are not my peeps. Women my age are my peeps, so I can help them make the most of their middle years.

Your shape is there, you just have to know how to go back to the beginning for it to come out again.

You need to put your Corset back on and lace the laces. It's not going to do you any good sitting in your drawer or unlaced.

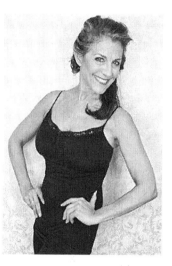

This program, *The 7 Secrets of a Sexy Silhouette*, and the online program to accompany this book, *The Corset and The Coat*, will re-familiarize your body on how you are designed to move. Why spend hours in the gym when you don't have to? You have grandchildren to enjoy and great adventures ahead of you, so find the juice!

Learn the secrets and start the whittling process to discover the treasures that already lie within and your body without hesitation or worry.

Unveil a personal Leonardo Da Vinci masterpiece unique to you, *a silhouette, confident and sexy.*

La Dolce Vita

Chapter One
Secret One

You have TWO cores
The Corset and the Coat

What is this inner core that lies deep within
It's called an inner Corset and sits beneath the skin
So let's pay attention and listen to what's in store
Your shape to return to hourglass, feel like 20 again and more
If there's one thing I have learned and I know you will surely see
Stay with me on this journey for a smaller waist, less pain, and less pee

"Without foundation, there can be no fashion."
Christian Dior

After 35 years as a fitness professional using my body one way, truly believing that I knew it all with regards to the core, in reality I knew everything about half of it, and it wasn't even the most important half! Why was I wearing myself out and leading others to do the same? I was training only what I saw and knew about; I literally had to stop everything I was doing and teaching overnight!

The reason we are losing our shape, have pain, or some other dysfunction is NOT because we have the wrong diet or don't exercise enough...that's only a piece of the puzzle.

It's because we have an inner core that isn't firing completely and sufficiently prior to the outer core. There's an order. The inside to the outside, its about timing.

The inner core gives you your shape, continence, and freedom of movement.

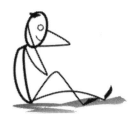 You have two cores and you have only been training one of them all these years, the outer core, the abdominals. These are the ones you can see and feel when you do a sit up or take a punch; these are the muscles on the outside, they are the wrapping, obliques, rectus abdominis, and sometimes the transverse abdominis. These are the outside or Coat muscles, the ones you have conscious control over and you can voluntarily train when you say you're going to do a bicep curl, or squat, sit up or Kegel, and you feel the muscle moving or tightening.

The inner core has the same muscle tissue, but is trained and functions in a completely different way. It resembles a capsule with a top and a bottom and sits inside the rib cage and pelvis.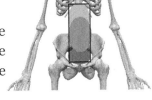

The top of the capsule is the diaphragm, the bottom is the pelvic floor, the front is the transverses abdominis, and the back and side are thoracolumbar fascia.

In anticipation of movement, your brain prepares your body.

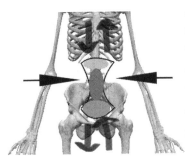 A millisecond prior to your actual movement, whether it's a cough or a walk, or merely picking up your coffee cup, the inner core gets a signal from the brain to fire all together at once to compress and compact the internal organs around the spine, stabilizing and protecting it prior to moving. This not

only frees up your periphery or mobility muscles for injury-free movement, but keeps internal organs propped, maintaining function!

These are your inner core muscles, your Corset. We call it a Corset because a Corset in its most general and original sense of the word is a garment that is worn right under the breast, lifting the boobs out of the way and down to the hip bones, compressing and holding that area stable. However, it wasn't just the compression, it also ordered your body in a certain way to support 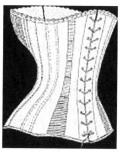 your back and of course is also a 'foundation' garment. This is the area we will be working on.

So you put on the Corset and then the clothes on top, which are the outer Coat muscles.

The Corset is not in our conscious awareness, it's an involuntary group of muscles; therefore, you don't train it directly like a bicep or tricep, like a Coat muscle, it must be triggered and allowed to fire prior to moving your outer core or voluntary periphery muscles.

The Corset is better trained with intention and imagery.

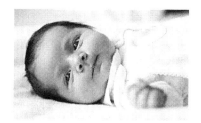 When babies are born they can't do anything. It takes a whole year of constant and progressive movement and the desire to get up and explore the world before they can get upright and continent. It's part of the developmental process; we had to constantly defy gravity because we kept falling down. The body had to get upright and stabilize. Before we could move our limbs independently and have freedom of movement on the outside, we had to have stability on the inside.

The inner core muscles are the stability muscles; they are what scooted you across the floor to get that shiny toy, without any arm or leg strength, and got you up on your feet to walk upright in the first place. You had no conscious control over your body. You didn't do squats, bicep curls, or Kegels to get off the ground. Nor do we need it today.

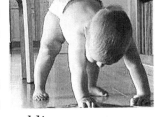

It was your inner core, then you became continent and could take off the diapers: this was your nervous system being wired in the world!

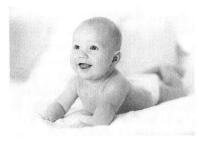

It's like this: a baby sees a toy she wants. In anticipation of getting that toy, an internal pressurization event happens, called Intra Abdominal Pressure, or IAP. It's like an internal fuselage that literally lifts her up. Her lungs fill with air, and the top of the Corset, the diaphragm, moves from a dome shape to a flattened pancake shape. This pushes the guts and organs downward towards the bottom of the Corset, the pelvic floor muscles. The pelvic floor muscles should respond to this increased pressure sort of like a trampoline, by catching, holding, *squeezing, and bouncing* the contents back up while the sides of the inner Corset simultaneously compress inward. This happens automatically to maintain a stable elongated spine so baby can balance her head on top and have a steady gaze for as long as possible.

Without stability in the inside, we are as helpless as a newborn. Then baby starts to develop and coordinate her outer voluntary muscles, the outer core, the Coat.

First the inner core prepares and compresses, then the outer core wraps and reinforces.

The Corset then the Coat.

Why doesn't it work anymore?

It's working, it's just weak unresponsive and fires in the wrong order, impairing function.

Many things can cause this.

Pregnancy, weight gain, inflammation, injury, illness, surgery—any of these can affect how you use your inner Corset. Even watching people who move incorrectly causes our brain to imitate those movement patterns and turn off or misfire our Corset. That's nature's way of wanting us to heal properly before we get up and move again. This internal program is still there, it's just asleep and activates late, after the outer Core or Coat muscles in response to a voluntary movement or conscious squeeze (we will talk later how visualization helps to get the appropriate order in Secret 4).

When the Corset doesn't pre-activate and fire before the Coat, you end up with problems, more injuries, low belly pooch, low back pain, hip pain, pelvic pain, urine leaks, hernias, prolapse, osteoporosis, bunions, spinal deviations, dysfunctional sex, thick thighs and ankles, and more because our amazing Corset activates and maintains our self-healing mechanisms.

We never learned to rehab our inner Corset correctly in the first place allowing them to neurologically reconnect, so they become glued together and instead, we go to the gym and train the voluntary muscles we can see, our Coat muscles to hold us still AND move us. We are pushing everything in from the outside. We get some shaping this way, but without a strong and responsive inner Corset or foundation, it's temporary and causes more health risks.

We start to develop compensations, which is like putting your foot on the gas and the brake at the same time--sort of pointless. And we get injured again, and go to the doctor and they tell us to go back to the gym or do Kegels or have surgery and keep training those voluntary Coat muscles, which is only making things worse, because we are doing it backwards.

It's all about TIMING. FIRST the inner core activates in anticipation of movement, SECOND The outer core then wraps and reinforces, IN THAT ORDER.

What everyone is doing in traditional training methods is training only the Coat muscle, which involves consciously thinking about it; like a sit-up, crunch, or Kegel, they're basically putting on their Coat or outer clothes on before their undergarments. It just doesn't work well that way.

Think of a suitcase. You can either just throw a big pile of clothes into the suitcase, stand on it, duct tape it, and pray that things don't drop out, or you can do it the orderly way. Fold, roll and compress the clothes, close the suitcase, and latch the latches. The very last you do is the duct tape or reinforcing.

Basically, all these years we have been just throwing a big pile of clothes into the suitcase and trying to duct tape it, praying things don't fall out, meaning we have been using our voluntary, or conscious muscles that we can feel to try to keep us all compacted and secure, stabilized and supported, when that's not the outer core's job.

We've been using our outer core muscles to do both jobs, to stabilize us and to mobilize us. No wonder we're getting injured and our body is not functioning properly.

Why doesn't my doctor know this?

Medicine is a fixing field, emphasizing injury and illness. It focuses on diagnosis and treatment of illness and injury, but you're not sick. You don't need a doctor. You just need to wake up your inner Corset so it starts working in the right order.

Medicine is undergoing a revolution; fitness is undergoing a revolution; but ultimately these people want you to pay them. I don't want you to pay me. I just want you to pay attention to this because you already have this inside your own body and you don't need to buy something new because you're not broken. I'm not talking about buying this book, because the secrets are priceless; it's not the same as buying a gadget. It's knowledge and doesn't feel like you're purchasing in the same way.

We cannot see the invisible Corset muscles, but those are the ones that really create the difference between a graceful dancer and a super athletic football player.

Those are the muscles that in pilates or yoga will transition your body gracefully from one pose to the other with stability, grace, and proper tension while holding it together. It's what you can't see that makes the difference, the inner Corset.

The Corset first compresses in anticipation of movement to stabilize and then the outer Coat layer wraps and reinforces, so we can move our limbs independently.

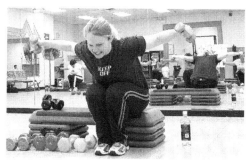

You can have many different Coats, but you only have one Corset. For instance, you can join different classes, join a gym, and do all kinds of exercises and have all different Coats, depending on what you want to do with your body, even be a bodybuilder--you can choose how you want to use your body. Those are all Coat exercises, but it isn't the exercises. The exercises are only the frosting on the cake. Who wants a cake with only frosting?

Ladies, take it from me, no matter how many sit ups, Pilates reformer classes, weight lifting competitions, or yoga workshops you do, the first thing you need to do is to get it out of your head that you need to train and squeeze from the outside to have a shape.

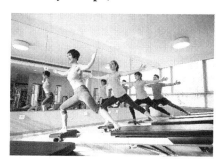

How can we as access the sleeping Corset?

Turn off the Coat muscles, then wake them up by rebooting the nervous system using imagery and intention.

It's the intention and image or picture that you have in your mind that fires your inner Corset.

It fires all in one piece prior to the outer Coat or voluntary muscles to stabilize and free up your outer core, your mobility muscles.

It's truly amazing how just by thinking of these images it reboots your brain and you won't have to think about it anymore. Just like you don't think about when you have to go somewhere how many steps it takes you to get there, you will just be able to focus on what you want to do and your brain will put all the correct steps in place.

You've already done it once as a baby; your body hasn't forgotten, we are going to just "wake it up," so it starts responding in a timely manner.

As you go through the exercises you may think, wow, it made sense as soon as you said it! I could feel it in my body!

The reason you can feel it in your body is because it's the way you learned how to move in the first place, so you've already done it.

You cannot work on your undergarments if you have your over garments on. Why put your underwear on the outside? You have to get rid of the Coat, to access your Corset.

The Corset is activated over and over, as long as you stop making it happen and reboot the system, then it will start to happen automatically, the same way you did when you were a child. You won't have to think about doing it anymore; it will become automatic and your Corset will be trained.

We have to go back to being a baby, so to speak. To access our Corset, we have to turn off our Coat muscles and train our awareness. We look at the inside and what's invisible by using visual imagery with intention while practicing simple movements, especially regular everyday type of movements.

I know you might not quite understand all of this right now, but you wouldn't have been able to learn how to walk without firing your inner Corset. No one taught you how to walk; the information is in there, in your brain; it just needs to be re-activated. The inner Corset and pelvic floor are automatically and consistently supporting, encapsulating, and compressing your organs, packing them and increasing disc space while keeping your body upright and strong.

If the inner Corset doesn't pre-activate, the added pressure of even something as simple as singing can be too much, and we can start to leak, or the organs begin to push through down towards the pelvic floor, causing issues.

When you start this program, it's just like a person who puts a Corset on for the first time; at first you can't lace it very tight and after a while the body gets trained and will get used to it. So, no worries.

> **Note:** As you go through the brain exercises it this book, it will feel like you're not doing ANYTHING. Don't worry, you are. It's just that your not used to activating this part of your brain, your imagination. Keep practicing, it gets easier.

> **Note:** Dr. Theresa suggests to in order to have a brain changing effect, three things to remember as you go through the exercises.

Mindfulness —a particular kind of focus — a new way of looking at something that tells your brain this is important and to pay attention, it will signal the brain that it's worth making new Mylan for (the insulation that makes the pathways go faster).

Movement — begins in your brain first with the image, activate your imagination and keep the Coat muscles turned off.

Mood — maintain a happy mood. In other words, you should not experience pain anywhere, as you go through these exercises. Even if your feeling noxious. Stop and start again.

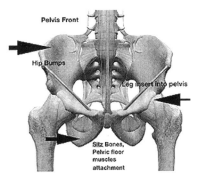

Let's start with a tour of the bones of the pelvis, because that's where your pelvic floor muscles attach, and how we will trigger the Corset. The pelvis is a big bony structure; your spine connects to it through the sacrum. The area of the pelvis that will also help activate the Corset are the Sitz bones. It's the same as the bones you sit on. You can feel it by reaching back or sitting on your hands; it's the two, sharp pointy things on each side of your crack, kind of where

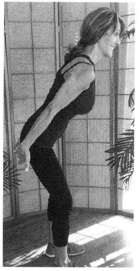

the outer edge of a kotex pad would be. When you sit, you should always be sitting on your Sitz bones, not your legs or your sacrum, which is where all the nerves are, most people are sitting on their nerves all day, meaning back pain.

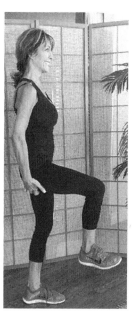

Now, stand up. The front bowl of the pelvis are the hip bumps or ridges, where you can hook your fingers. The hip socket underneath is where your legs hook in, fist width apart and half way back.

So now point to the Sitz bones and lift your knee like a marionette, without swinging and bringing it up with your butt. The leg socket is a big strong joint. Notice when you lift your thigh, the Sitz bone is lower than your leg. So, your torso goes all the way to the bottom of the pelvis. Your legs are not part of your torso.

So, when you bend, don't bend at your low back, that's not the middle of you. Bend at the underwear line. Put your hands and make a karate chop and send the Sitz bones back. The spine moves in one piece, and that is the middle of you.

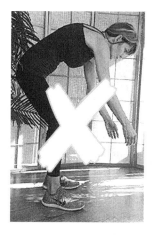
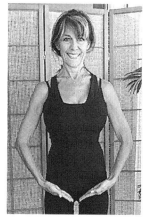
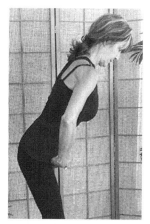

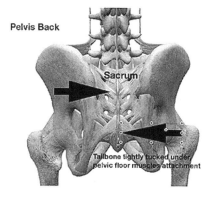

Pelvis Back

Sacrum

Tailbone tightly tucked under pelvic floor muscles attachment

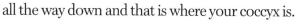

At the end of the spine is a tiny bone called the coccyx, or tailbone. Put your hand on your sacrum, take your middle finger and put it at the top of your butt crack and follow the tip of your middle finger all the way down and that is where your coccyx is.

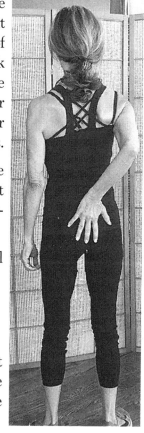

The coccyx has some ability to move and the great thing is the pelvic floor muscles connect to the coccyx. When we even imagine it moving, it still triggers the pelvic floor/Corset.

When we activate any part of the Corset, it all activates together, simultaneously.

Activate your Corset to sit in your chair.

Parasol — Guts before Butts

Remember, it's the picture in your mind that triggers the pelvic floor, the Corset. The more you practice activating your imagination the better the results!

Your guts are heavy and they sit in the pelvic bowl. There's no air in there only guts, they are the packing peanuts, always packing around our spine and pushing down on the pelvic floor.

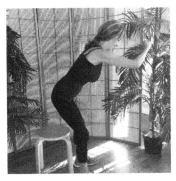

An upside down Parasol is shaped the same way as the pelvic bowl, it sits inside and has a handle. The handle is your spine and is directed forward.

Before you sit, hold onto this handle and literally feel like you can pull up on it.

When you pull up on the handle, it lifts those heavy guts and then you can send your sitz bones back and sit. Don't tighten the legs or the tummy, just send the sitz bones back and sit on them. It also works in reverse to get out of a chair. Use it also to climbing stairs or walk up a hill.

So now let's turn off the Coat Muscles, the ones we can see and consciously feel.

Mr. Freeze — Understanding the difference between tension and relaxation

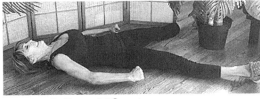

Lay down on the ground and tense every muscle in your body like you're frozen and stiff for a few seconds. Do you feel that tension? Great! That is your outer core or Coat muscles that you can voluntarily squeeze at will.

Now release the tension. Let your butt go, belly go, everything. Imagine your muscles are melting off your bones into the ground like warm butter. Do you 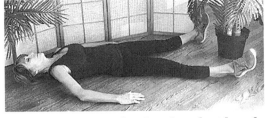 feel that? Great, you should feel nothing, completely relaxed with only your brain working. You are taking off your Coat to access the Corset.

Chapter Two
Secret Two

Why Kegels Don't Cut It
There's No Core Without the Floor

When I cough and when I sneeze I feel a little spritz

Needless to say it's stressful this way like my body's on the fritz

I'm excited to say, there is another way, so how can I keep from speaking

At this age and stage of life, there's more laughing, more loving, and less leaking.

Marie, 48, is a physical therapist who came to a one-hour presentation I did for 30 medical providers on the inner Corset a few years ago. She called me a few days later and told me that she has been leaking urine when she coughs or sneezes for the last few years, and she's never had kids! Kegels weren't working, and it was getting worse until she came to my presentation. Surprised that just the Reed exercise could stop her leaks literally overnight, she signed up for sessions and went back and re-educated all of her patients.

Today she says, "Reversing my patterns has been huge. I can stand, walk, and bend with much more safety and confidence. My leaking is gone and I won't be needing a hip replacement or spinal fusion surgery! I cannot adequately express the positive impact this work has had on my body and my long-term prognosis."

The pelvic floor is the bottom of the Corset and there is no core without the Floor!

Do you wonder why Kegels don't quite cut it anymore?

It is because there are three layers of the pelvic floor, not one. The Kegel layer is NOT meant to hold back the pee, OR keep your internal organs propped.

I loved it when Dr. Theresa explained how the pelvic floor layers are like a shoe.

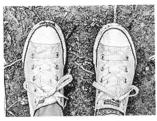

It really helped me make a picture in my mind and hopefully it will help you too. Think of your bare foot in the shoe itself. The sole is the strongest part of the shoe; it surrounds and supports your foot. This is like the innermost and strongest layer of the pelvic floor. If the shoe is worn out and gets a rip or a tear, you have a big problem because you won't even HAVE a shoe. No support at all.

The middle is quite different in men and women. The muscle tissue in both runs from side to side, like the laces on the shoe. They can be very tight and painful with a lot of muscular tension or very loose with no tension at all, because the laces loosen when you take your shoe off, when you have a baby. When you put your shoe back on, you should bring your laces back together again—the nervous system should reboot and bring the connection back, but for a lot of women they stay separated.

These two layers are the most important layers of the pelvic floor, but they are not in our conscious awareness. These two layers are part of the inner Corset; the floor of the core; they are supposed to pre-activate before the outer Kegel or Coat muscle.

The Kegel layer is the bow on the shoe. That's the layer we usually work on: it has millions and millions of nerve endings because this is where our conscious continence takes place--it's the faucet. We can feel it when we cut off a stream of urine, and we feel the tightening when we do it.

The Kegel muscle and sphincters are the outer layers of the pelvic floor; they are all part of the Coat. You are aware of them, you can feel them, but they are outside muscles like the abdominal muscles. Think of Kegels as like the abs of your "hoochie."

Because there are millions of nerves, we think we are doing a whole lot, but we're actually trying to use something very flimsy to try and fix something substantial.

We're not aware of the 30-40 pounds of weight in our guts. We are more aware of the fat in our belly then we are of the weight in our guts that pushes down.

Don't get me wrong, it's not that Kegels are bad, it's just that they are not enough.

As we age, shoes that used to be sturdy, reliable shoes turn into something that's a lot flimsier. But they can still work. Even if they are thin, they still surround and support your foot.

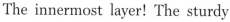

Your guts and internal organs weigh 30 to 40 pounds, so what the heck is holding them up from falling out of the bottom of your body? That's a lot of weight, that's not one bowling ball but a couple of bowling balls.

The innermost layer! The sturdy part the of the shoe, the one that does the heavy lifting, and has the highest resting tone in the body. Sometimes we compare it with a trampoline because when it's working well and the guts get pushed down, this layer will always push everything back up, because it fires along with the rest of the Corset, constantly stabilizing.

How the pelvic floor should work:

Think of the guts and the downward pressure like an upside-down tube of toothpaste. What would happen if you had a loose lid? Nothing is going to run out, The tube is supposed to be holding the toothpaste, even if the lid is barely on, but if you squeeze the tube of toothpaste, it's going to squirt out. The point is, the innermost layers of the pelvic floor, the laces that pull the shoe together, are supposed to respond and take the pressure off the outer layer, the Kegel, the bow.

Think of the Kegel as the dam behind the dam, the fire hydrant behind the faucet. Behind the faucet (Kegel) is the water pressure. The water pressure cannot overwhelm your faucet, otherwise water will get all over your kitchen floor.

It isn't the Kegel or faucet that keeps the water back; the water main keeps the water back, which is the strongest and most supportive innermost trampoline layer and allows the water to come in as the faucet turns on and off as needed, which is the Kegel layer.

You can't control the fire hydrant amount of water pressure with the faucet. You have to have something in between. The other pelvic floor layers are in between and should work and exist as part of the inner Corset. They fire all at one time, taking the pressure off the Kegel layer, the bow.

One of the reasons we shouldn't pee when we cough is because our brain knows a microsecond before we cough, It lifts and tones the entire pelvic floor in the correct sequence, moving it up and away and then reinforcing right before the pressure increases from the cough.

This happens in anticipation of that pressure. The pelvic floor lifts so that the whole thing doesn't blow through like a toothpaste tube with a loose cap.

When you cough or laugh, the pushing down of the guts is what pushes on the weakened pelvic floor, which overwhelm the Kegel layer, the bow.

Even if you're not aware that you're about to cough or sneeze, it's the anticipation that the pelvic floor tones by lifting the guts away, so the gut weight doesn't press down and overwhelm the faucet, which is how the Kegel muscle works.

Doing Kegels is like turning the faucet on and off or repairing the faucet. But the problem is not the faucet at all; the problem is much bigger than the faucet.

It's not that the faucet or Kegel isn't important. It's just the part we can see inside our house but is also very important to be aware of what goes on behind it.

We have a continent threshold. When we were younger, we not only had more youthful tissue tone down there, but we didn't weigh or cough as much as we do now.

For instance, if someone tickles you and you laugh hysterically, or if you jump on a trampoline, you leak. It's called stress incontinence. It's the amount of stress needed to cause incontinence, which is usually a spritz or spurt. I'm not talking about urge incontinence, where you go all at once. In that instance, the neurological signal from the brain turned off the continent mechanism and you start to pee like a man and you can't stop once you start. I'm not talking about that one, although it is helped by this program. In this book, I refer to stress incontinence.

When we are older, we have more pressures on the pelvic floor. It's either stretched out or damaged from years ago and was never properly rehabilitated. Instead we do Kegels, which worked for a while but now with the added stress to the tissue, either the Kegel muscle isn't working, or the pressure has increased, or the other two innermost layers of at the pelvic floor, the strongest layers, are not doing anything to unburden the outer Kegel layer.

We start to experience more problems of holding our bladder. But this is a symptom of overall non-functioning of the inner Corset.

When the Corset is unresponsive (the laces on the shoe are too loose or too tight) and doesn't respond by lifting and supporting the guts, but instead allow the pressure of the guts to push down on the vulnerable outer flimsy Kegel layer, this will eventually overcome the ability of the faucet to contain at least a small bit of the urine, so it will squirt out from too much pressure.

The toothpaste won't come out of the tube unless you squeeze it. You need the extra squeeze that comes from bearing down, coughing, jumping, or just doing something.

For some women, the pelvic floor can be so stretched out they even have problems with the reproductive organs descending towards outside of the body, called prolapse.

It's just turned off and we have been using more duct tape or the outer reinforcement layers, like the Kegel muscle, to hold everything up and in; it's exhausting and pointless.

It's like picking up a cantaloupe with dental floss. By only doing Kegels and trying to catch everything on this little tiny muscle, there's no security and things are falling out in many directions.

We keep doing Kegels over and over, because it's the only part of the pelvic floor that we are aware of and can feel and can consciously control; because it's so full of nerve endings you think you're doing a lot, but it's not going to hold your shoe in place if your laces are undone and if your shoe is flapping.

Your shoe needs to be repaired.

The laces have to be tied not too tight or too loose, and then you can tie the bow, Kegel. You can practice tying the bow, but it's not going to help you hold your shoe in place unless all the other layers are done first.

So not only is everything falling out of the bottom, it's also exploding out to the sides, which is causing you to lose your waistline because the laces aren't in place. Your ribs are flaring and the stomach is pooching. The whole thing is turned off and we have to turn it back on; so we're going to learn how to flip the internal switch for proper lacing.

When the pelvic floor and whole internal Corset function like it's supposed to, besides less leaking, you will have also sculpted a shape from the armpits to the bottom of your torso.

The Kegel is not designed to hold up the whole shoe, or all that pressure. If you force it to do that job, it's not surprising that after years and years of overuse and abuse it finally says 'I'm done with you. I'm not even going to do what I can do." So you keep coaxing it and it doesn't work anymore. To make this problem even worse, when women go into menopause or the midlife hormonal changes happen, a decrease in estrogen happens, which makes the tissues even thinner.

We have turned off both the laces, and the most important part of the pelvic floor, the innermost, strongest, and most supportive part of the shoe, without making it tone.

The innermost layer is now flimsy, out of use and non-responsive; the middle layer is unlaced during childbirth to accommodate the delivery of a child and then failed to rehabilitate properly to bring the laces back together. So we never get off the baby weight and can't get the waistline back; because we stopped having good function of the pelvic floor, we keep adding to the burdens over time and it progressively gets worse and worse.

The Good News

We can access these deep pelvic floor layers because it connects to the Kegel outer layers. We can go through the faucet and back through the plumbing and find out where the working parts are and access way up there even though we can't see.

Since the three layers are all attached together with a little French knot at the perineum, when we train the innermost strongest layer, the other two layers come along for the ride in the correct sequential order of firing from inside to outside.

This will allow your Kegel muscle to properly perform its job, which is to start and stop the flow, the faucet, and sexual function which we will discuss in Secret Sex, I mean Secret Six.

Down Under

Some women are not aware they have three different openings down there. Each of these holes are surrounded by muscle, a squeeze muscle that you have conscious control over. The bow, reinforcement layer, and abs of your hoochie are the ones that you have conscious control over.

The front is the urethra near the pubic bone. You can squeeze and stop the flow of urine.

The middle is the vagina where you put a tampon. You can tighten it. It's where the baby comes out and where you have sex. It's not a ring but more of a cuff, a whole hand cuff. It surrounds and encompasses the penis. Women tend to have a lax middle layer from the hormones of pregnancy to let the baby out or take the shoe off. We want the cuff to be working without turning on the outer Coat muscles. What happens with some women and a lot of men is that the middle layer of the pelvic floor becomes very tight and tense because of the outer Coat squeeze (by tensing butt and doing Kegels).

The muscle around the anus is a sphincter, we call it the Winky. This muscle has to release to have a bowel movement and pass gas, so It needs to know right away what's coming out—air, liquid, or firm. Then it knows how much to open up the faucet, a tiny bit, medium or wide. It's the smartest of the sphincters, because it has to be able to sense what's sitting behind the door or behind the crack.

Women will do a Kegel, stop the flow and do the tampon exercise where you try to pull an imaginary tampon up higher into your vagina like an elevator, up up up. But what women are really doing is clenching all their other muscles and using the butt muscles to push the elevator or tampon up.

There's a better way!

We need to stop Kegeling and learn to let go, otherwise it won't get better, because we need to access the innermost pelvic floor layer. You can't do it by Kegeling or clenching your butt cheeks all the time. That's what causes that dent in the derrière, it's from clenching all the time, which is pulling on the laces really hard, making for a tight laces and more back pain.

When our Corset turns off to have a baby, surgery, illness, it will stop firing in a timely manner because the nerves didn't relearn in time to bring the laces back together.

That's why we use nervous system training in this program, not muscular training. It's not the muscle isn't strong enough or that it's not connected the right way with the nervous system, it's that it's asleep and it has not been called on to help support the guts.

The way to train the innermost pelvic floor layers is just like a nerve muscle connection, which trains both the nervous system and the muscle at the same time--imagery and visualization.

When we use imagery, we can also turn off our Coat.

When we move the bony landmarks of the pelvic floor (Sitz bones, tailbone), where the muscles attach, it tugs on these muscles of the pelvic floor like the shoe. Like when you move your foot in the shoe you affect the leather on the shoe, the most supportive part. If you move the bony landmarks where the muscles attach it will actually pull on them and start to wake them up. Even if we just think about moving the tail bone and Sitz bones, it will activate the pelvic floor and the whole Corset.

The brain thinks they are not doing anything, so imagery helps us send messages from the brain to the pelvic floor by tugging on the pelvic floor from moving other parts that directly touch it. This sends messages from the pelvic floor back to the brain. The messages need to go in both directions like a telephone line; it needs to be like dialogue. As messages go back, more messages come out.

Even tiny little movements can result in a big bang with your nervous system.

Since the innermost layers are part of the inner Corset, we can't train them like a Kegel contraction you can feel. It's like the rest of the Corset, it must be triggered and allowed to activate.

The first thing we have to do is learn how to turn off these outer tight muscles. That may sound strange, but most women hold themselves in some kind of tension all day long.

EXERCISES

Let's first identify the Coat muscles of the pelvic floor that we will be turning off.

Lie down and do a Kegel, pull up, like you're stopping the flow of pee. Now pretend you have a tampon in and your you're pulling it up further through your vagina. Now pull up on your anus or butt hole muscle, like you're trying to hold back passing gas at a party, the Winky muscle. These are Coat muscles.

Now that you know, let's stay away from doing those until we can access the innermost strongest trampoline layer and learn the correct sequence.

Exercise

LAY AN EGG – Releases the outer layers to access the innermost layer and wake it up.

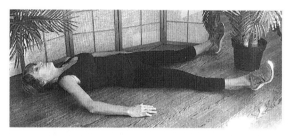

Sit or lay down and imagine you're a chicken and lay an egg out of your anus—that's right, no pushing. Just allow it to come out. Did you know chickens cannot lay eggs when they're stressed? Let it just come out. Lay one, two or a few.

Activate the Corset

THE REED – The cornerstone exercise of this program, we literally activate the brain and nervous system and start training those connections that pull and tug the strongest layer of the pelvic floor, which is going to 'wake it up' making more nerves, increasing blood flow, muscle tone and removal of toxic waste.

For over two thousand years, Yogis have practiced an advanced technique to become a master. They knew there was a place deep inside that gave them health, wellness, lightness, and freedom of movement. When practicing the final test to be a Yogi Master, they took a reed, a straw-like hollow tube that grows in the water. They inserted it up their rectum or Winky, as we call it, and would suck water very high up, while keeping the anus, Winky, relaxed.

Don't worry, in our case, we will just practice being a Yogi Master. We won't actually put a reed up our butt. But, by using our imagination with the Reed, we are literally activating things, so we are going to imagine this without pinching off the end. When you watch a child first suck through a straw, notice how they tend to pinch the end off with their lips. This is important for us to know as we practice the Reed image. It's important that we DON'T pinch off at the end with the Winky. No clenching of the butt muscles. They must stay turned off.

Sit on your Sitz bones or lie down and imagine a small steam of water is going up through the Reed high up the back passage. Sip, sip, sip; then the water bounces up, like a Bingo or Lotto Ball. Up, up, up; up an inch, then down an inch, up an inch and a half, down and inch, up two inches, down an inch... always keeping the bingo or lotto ball bouncy feeling way up high

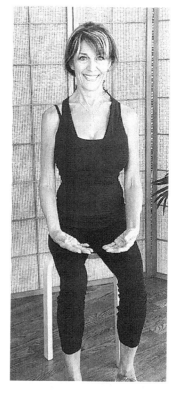

in your rectum. It's like there's a constant stream of water always moving up this Reed. There is a sensation of keeping everything relaxed and creating a bubbly internal feeling of things moving up. The key for you is to visualize.

When you first start with this image, everything will begin to twitch and want to help out, like your Winky or butt, that's okay, just stop, Lay an Egg and try again. Your body is trying to accomplish something, which is lift the water up. Stillness and calm is what's important and not trying to help out all the time. If you try to sense it, that means you're trying to do it. The key is not to try and do it but imagine what it would be like without moving another single muscle in your whole body. The trick is the only thing moving is your mind. Everything else is turned off. You might feel it in the ears or the roof of your mouth or back of nose and head. This is where the suction is created. Pay attention to your butt. Is it still turned on? Practice letting it go; keep practicing letting it go while maintaining the Reed.

You need to keep that feeling of suction. Vacuum the intensity up inside. Relax butt and Winky. No pushing or pulling.

Practice the Reed 24/7, or as much you can, when your walking, reading a book, lifting a coffee cup, doing dishes, watching TV, laying down and with all the other exercises. Soon it will be automatic.

The Reed poem

Mr Reed Mr Reed, I thank God every day for you

I feel light on my feet again when I did not know what to do

You have kept me from leaking flattened my tummy and kept my organs from falling

Corrected my posture cured my depression to keep me from every day bawling

Even though you're just a stream of water running up my rectum towards my ears

Just imagining you throughout the day I haven't felt this good in years!

BIKINI BREATHING

Now we are going to learn how to increase the Intra Abdominal Pressure, IAP, that triggers the baby mechanism, the Corset that got us up to walk in the first place.

A baby always does things in the correct order.

At birth, nothing. Then they look, roll over, sit up, crawl, walk, run, and jump. Each time the Corset (inner core) pre-activates it gets stronger, then the baby can keep developing the outer core, Coat muscles. They can't lift their body up until they can lift their pelvic floor up. It's the last part of the Corset to develop, that's why jumping is the very last thing we are able to do.

Now, let's go back and remind ourselves what we went through to get prepared for learning how to walk.

We turned off our Coat, now we will understand how our ribs move.

The main thing is to always keep the ribs soft and downward. They have to stay down in the same position that you feel when you blow up a balloon or exhale maximally, all the time.

Breathe in and breathe out maximally. When the ribs are dropped down and not allowed to lift, and you don't move anything else, and breathe in, you will increase the IAP, a GOOD thing, because the ribs are not expanding in the front, maybe a tad on the sides.

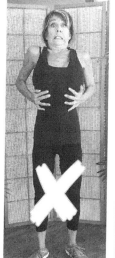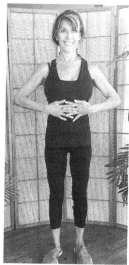

Breathe in, and you feel the ribs open to a Sunrise, and then you want to close them into Sunset with the full exhalation and keep them closed, to activate your Corset.

Imagine you're wearing a triangle bikini front and back. Put your hands on the bikini front, as you inhale, feel the air actually going into your bikini all the way around.

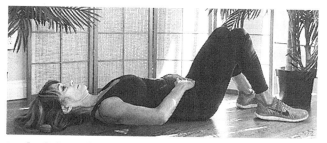

When you keep the ribs down in Sunset and breathe in, instead of the expansion going into your ribs, the expansion will be in the bikini front and back and will increase IAP.

Feel the air go down and expand your bikini front and back equally. We want to start to sense this inside pressurization that compresses and compacts everything all secure around our spine; this is the baby mechanism that gets them up onto their feet.

Note: If your bikini is not expanding but collapsing under your

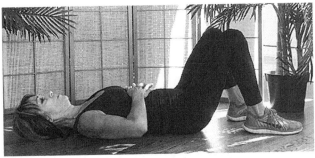

fingers, put your hands back on your ribs to help keep them down until you can maintain Sunset position. If you feel your ribs lifting to breathe, you are probably sucking your stomach in, so no sucking your tummy in or no clenching of your butt. You will also learn to turn off your Coat muscles by learning to breathe correctly. If you notice your belly, back, face, or neck tensing, release, stop, and do Mr. Freeze. Then blow up an imaginary balloon to get the ribs softly into Sunset or exhale maximally.

When lying down, always maintain Sunset ribs and a small space under your low back, enough space for an imaginary sleeping butterfly. So you must never push your low back down. Feet underneath knees, toes slightly turned out.

Keep practicing with Sunset to increase the IAP to activate or trigger our Corset, with the Reed exercise. Eventually you won't have to think about it anymore, and could be as soon as today. That's how fast the nervous system can reboot!

SITZ BONES WALKING

Turn your tight hard or floppy flaccid pelvic floor muscles into a springy lively pelvic floor that holds up your guts and pulls in your Corset.

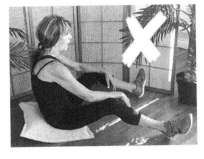

First, sit on your Sitz bones, make sure you're not sitting on your sacrum.

Sit on the floor, or on a pillow or stack of books, to help get up on the Sitz bones. Legs in a V, and bent, don't straighten the legs. In front of you there's an imaginary handle on the floor that's literally

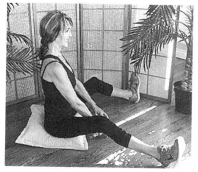

cemented into the floor and you can you literally use your fingers on the handle to rotate your pubic bone down and back to get the Sitz bones on the ground.

Now, tack down the right Sitz bone, and lift the left one stretching it up and away and tack it down. Then pick up the other side literally walking forward.

Do this exercise when you're watching TV hanging out or doing nothing at all because every time you walk with one Sitz bone versus the other you're stretching and pulling on the pelvic floor and turn your pelvic floor into something a whole lot more!

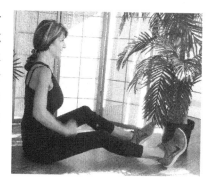

Continence and mobility

There's a quarter of the bones of the body in your feet. That means lots of joints and one of the biggest and strongest triggers to your inner Corset is what happens when your foot touches the ground. If you have a stiff or tense foot, the pelvic floor is not responding properly and not elevating.

The arches of the foot and the pelvic floor are wired together in your brain, When the arches of your foot started to develop after about 18 months or so after you got up to walk, that was the same time to remove diapers.

So whatever is going on with our feet will affect our pelvic floor and whole inner Corset. Whatever's going on with our pelvic floor or inner Corset will affect our feet. If your feet are tense and stiff, you will have a tense and stiff pelvic floor. Likewise, if your feet are floppy and have no tension or tone in them, so will your pelvic floor. If you work on one, the other improves. In other words, if you do exercises for the inner Corset, your mobility will improve just the same as if you do this Plunger Foot exercise, your leaking or back pain will improve.

So we do this exercise to trigger the Corset.

PLUNGER FEET

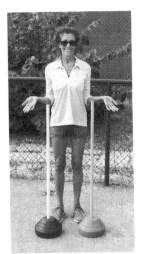

Stand with feet hip, fist width apart, toes wider than heels, knees unlocked.

Imagine your foot is a toilet plunger. The arch is the rubber thingy and your shin is the handle. Keep the ball of the foot in contact with the floor with the toes relaxed lengthening forward, imagine the heel bone directed diagonally back.

Use your shin, the handle, to splay the foot, as if the arches can go flat, and the bones spread, then lift from the handle and the arch or rubber thingy comes up, keeping the long toes and heels on the ground the whole time. Keep your butt soft, no clenching.

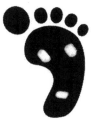

When you walk, walk on the tripod, the base of the big toe at the ball of the foot, fourth toe at the ball and base of heel at the same time, that means NO 'heel toe' heel toe' walking, it's more like you are plunging the arch of the foot, the rubber thingy, down and up, splaying the bones and springing them back up. Creating more space between the joints.

Squish, Squish, squish goes the Toilet Plunger Feet.

When you splay and spring, splay and spring it's another way to activate and strengthen your pelvic floor, the bottom of your inner Corset.

So let's go! Splay spring, splay, spring goes our toilet plunger feet.

I had no clue that in my shoe lived a foot that works like a plunger
I step forward, I step back, my arches squish down, up, from under
Splay and spring, splay and spring my arch is a suction cup
Heals down and back, toes long and relaxed, as the arch springs
down up down up.

Chapter Three
Secret Three

You Can't Out Exercise Your Desk Job
You're Not Where You Think You Are

We've been told to lose weight we must exercise

The latest science now proves otherwise,

You don't need exercise, just get lively and move more

Refine your general everyday movement to expedite the chore

First stop the cardio workouts to reduce the belly fat

We now know that it's a whole lot simpler than that

Then we update the brain's map for daily movement efficiency

To update our map, awareness and imagery is key

To reclaim your body for less pain and get your shape back

Realign your bones, put on your Corset, then your Coat after that.

Marcie is a Japanese Acupressure Therapist at Scripps Memorial Hospital La Jolla Cardiac Treatment Center in San Diego and came to my fitness class years ago held at the hospital. After class, she came up to me and complained about the shoulder pain she was having for quite some time. I gave her a Movement Mapping (TM) exercise that immediately took away her pain. A year later she injured herself and couldn't do the hard workouts anymore, wasn't losing any weight, only building mass and wasn't feeling good.

She came back to me and decided to stop working OUT and start working IN in order to reboot and reorganize.

Since then she has lost 20 pounds and feels better than ever.

"It's simple, it's all awareness and visualization techniques! I love this program!" says Marcie.

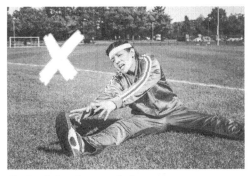

If you don't enjoy exercise as much as a dish of ice cream or a glass of wine, you might as well skip the workout, because it's just pointless.

There are over 30,000 gyms, workout fads, and even more diets out there, yet the bulge doesn't budge and there are even more repetitive injuries.

Then, we sit at a desk all day and say we're going to go exercise after work because we sat all day. It won't work because you've already set your hormones up to sabotage you, causing hormonal shifts (more so in women) and then we think we can go to the gym and out exercise our desk job?

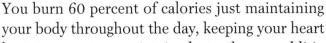

But the opposite is true. You burn more calories by the general everyday movement you do rather than the exercise.

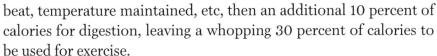

You burn 60 percent of calories just maintaining your body throughout the day, keeping your heart beat, temperature maintained, etc, then an additional 10 percent of calories for digestion, leaving a whopping 30 percent of calories to be used for exercise.

You also burn more calories sitting and daydreaming than watching TV and burn more calories taking a walk to visit a friend instead of just taking a walk.

The brain likes purposeful and intentional movement.

If it's not purposeful and intentional movement of daily living, it will create a lot more stress hormones which accumulate around your waist to protect fragile internal organs. Your brain is saying, "What the heck are you doing running on a rubber platform that goes round and round to nowhere land... there's isn't a tiger chasing you so, I'm not going to use this fat, I will store it around these fragile internal organs for protection...no tellin' what this maniac workout gal will do next!"

When we don't stop to rehab our inner Corset correctly, our brain, the GPS system, the control center for all movement, conscious and unconscious, will then recruit different Coat muscles that we keep training to take over and we become full of compensations, which is why we have pain and it hurts too much to move.

When the Corset fires in a timely manner prior to the Coat, it pulls everything together from the inside, joints automatically line up for less injury and it frees up your periphery muscles arms and legs; you won't have to think about positioning your body to move, when your Corset is rebooted. It's called Dynamic Joint Centration.

Making a movement is like having a hotline to your brain wiring things in place. But because of the compensations, we have stopped moving things we didn't even know existed and our body is getting frozen.

When a muscle is not moving properly contracting and releasing, the brain literally puts scar tissue in the muscle, turning it into more like a piece of canvas, a tissue that doesn't have any give, just stiff and hard with a strap to hold it there all the time, until you move it again.

So we are stiff and tense and we trot on down to the massage therapist who says we're tight, and they massage it out until next time. But what you may not know is that it's your brain keeping everything tight. Our muscles can control movement, but they are always listening to a brain that wants to protect us from injury.

Our brain is set to avoid particular kinds of injuries and has been for millions of years so it will set us up for protection. If someone asked why can't you do the Chinese splits, you tell them you actually can! There's nothing that connects the two legs. When your brain is turned off with anesthesia, doctors can move your body in any way they want. So why does it require continuous training to practice the Chinese splits? Because your brain doesn't like you in these precarious positions where the movement has no purpose and you would be prone to injury.

We want to be able to move wherever and however we want without worry.

It's like taking the most efficient route to work, which happens to be over the bridge. One day the bridge collapsed, (you have an injury) so you had to find another route to get there, (a compensation develops, such as leaning to one side or still waddling from a previous pregnancy) which happens to be the long way around, meaning more wear and tear on your car, burning more gas and more trips to the mechanic; but you still get there, eventually.

Finally, the bridge gets fixed, (your injury healed) but you were so used to the road and the trips to the mechanic you never thought it was possible that you even COULD go back over that bridge.

Translation, we get better but our compensations (Coat muscles) have already taken control and now fighting for complete control.

Movement therapies in the last 50 years involve working with our outer Coat muscles, the voluntary muscles, the ones we can tense up and feel, like a bicep. It's easy to create multiple compensations and become stiff and tense like a Lego man, frozen, barely able to move anymore.

We all have to get older but we can maintain lots of usefulness and move our body in a way that's offers less stress and strain.

We want to be less stiff and tense, we want to be more like a Neiman Marcus version of a robot with many moving parts always signaling back and forth to the mainframe computer. We want to move with graceful effortless efficiency, where movement is refined and we don't have to think about it anymore.

Since exercise can be stressful or stress relieving and we lack general everyday purposeful movement and most of our calories are burned by the general movement we do DURING the day rather than the actual exercise, it makes more sense to refine general movements to decrease stress, and ultimately belly fat accumulation.

I am talking about refining everyday unconscious movement, movement that we don't really think about.

So along with rebooting the Corset, we also will update our brain/GPS with Movement Mapping™another program Invented by Dr. Theresa. It takes the guess work out of how to move.

When we go to move a muscle, like doing a bicep curl, it signals the brain to move the joint, indirectly.

A faster and more direct way to move a muscle is to focus on the joint with Movement Mapping™ This will recalibrate and hardwire the brain so you won't have to think about how to move anymore.

You can start going back over that bridge again and save money on gas, the mechanic and wear and tear on your car and you didn't even know you could!

Movement Mapping™ is a neuro-based program for daily movement efficiency.

The goal of Movement Mapping™ is to develop anatomy awareness. We do this by telling your brain how your body is organized and to experience a better, more efficient way to move. Poor mapping can cause a lot of tension and strain due to these compensatory movements. Movement Mapping™ updates the brain's map of where the joints are, reorganizing creating automatic efficiency of movement.

We do this by awareness exercises and by moving the joint without including the muscles using imagery. Since the outside of us doesn't look like the inside of us, sometimes we will have a wrong picture of where our joints are; so we need to update our GPS (brain) so our body, the map, doesn't keep running off the side of the road, (repetitive injuries).

This kind of movement, Movement Mapping™, the smaller movement, changes the way you feel all the time. Not just after a workout… ugh, I remember those days I couldn't wait for my jog to finish so I could go home and eat something decadent.

So, ladies, you don't have to exercise and by all means skip the cardio if you're not enjoying it as much as a glass of wine. Sit less, get lively, and move more, and understand the general principles of movement as well as the skills of eating in Evolutionary Eating.

Increase fat burning by doing Hi Intensity Interval Training (HIIT) for short periods of time. HIIT burns a lot more calories, takes a lot less time, and keeps your body tuned up. Try jump rope or hopscotch. Work up to 20 seconds of all out Intensity and 10 second break for 10-20 minutes, 3-4 times a week. Start with what you can do safely and work up.

EXERCISES – key words that tell the brain how the body is organized.

APPLE CORE

A big problem we have that contributes to people with back pain is they think their spine is behind them like a thin broomstick. We have been told for many years to stand up straight and pull our shoulders back, and again we have Coat muscles trying to hold us up the best way possible, but we do it in the wrong place, from the back.

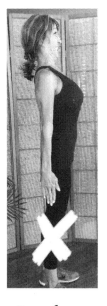

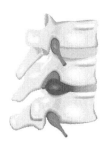 When we stand this way we will crimp the spinal processes that are narrow and where the nerves come out in the back, so when you stand up straight and stack up from the back, you're chronically crushing the nerves roots as they come out.

And when you squeeze your shoulder blades together it sends your head forward, throwing alignment off, adding to further back pain. There's no straightening or squeezing.

The most supportive, largest, and most weight-bearing part of your spine is in the middle and in the front, behind your belly button. The spine starts behind your eyes between your ears, curves toward your belly button, inserts through the pelvis at the sacrum, and ends at the coccyx.

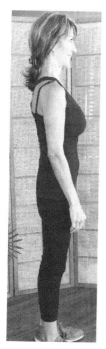

We want to feel our body stacked more towards the front and then we have more freedom in the back. This is what we call Apple Core.

Your spine runs through you and there is as much on the back of you as the front of you.

Imagine you are an Apple Core, with no outer core tension. Think about this image when you're walking and when you're sitting. No stiffening, straightening or squeezing of the Coat muscles.

TOOTSIE POP HEAD

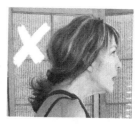

Your head sits on top of your spine, like a Tootsie Pop. Half of your skull is behind you and your face is in front. Allow your

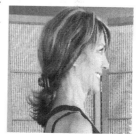

mouth to slightly open and jaw is relaxed. Your tongue is at the roof or dome of your mouth with the tip of the tongue behind your front teeth on the steps without touching the back of the front teeth.

HANGER to reclaim collar bones.

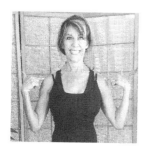

Imagine the little shelf where our arms hang down are as far apart as they can be. The line from the ears to the top of the shoulders where a general would wear his epaulets, is as long as it can be. Imagine both lines are as long

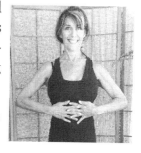

as they can be.

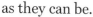

Put your hand on your collar bones and move them up and down a few times.

The collarbones are attached to the scapula which are shaped like triangles. If you move your collarbone forward your scapula moves forward, when you move your collarbones up and down, and forward back your scapula moves. Your shoulder blades are like a little cape, they glide along your rib cage. Your rib cage is circular and your scapula should feel like triangular pieces of buttered bread that move over the back surface.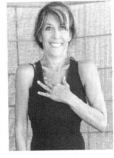

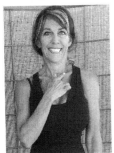

Your arms are attached on the front of the rib cage, like a whip handle, and your arm is the whip.

The whip handle can move in little circles or big circles and the arms follow and you have a whip.

SNOWMAN will help you get a sense of your spine alignment so that each section of your torso and head is placed in the proper balanced position, which means your Corset can be fully activated

The bottom ball is the bowl of the pelvis, then the rib cage which is rounded aligns directly over. Then your head is the top ball. Imagine Tootsie Pop Head without any tension.

STACKING WITH SPACE – Kiss and Tell

Since our bodies are frozen, we are walking around all stiff and tense like a Lego man and everything is stuck together, like our joints, so we need to separate them and make space. It's called Kiss and Tell. We do this by compressing the joint, then releasing the joint, same idea when we do Toilet Plunger Feet and the splay and spring action with compression and release.

Stand, maintain alignment, Sunset ribs, Snowman and Hanger. Imagine you can make space inside of you from the ground up.

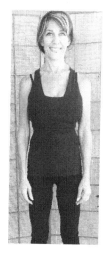 Activate your Toilet Plunger Feet creating space from the ground up through the arch, under the ankle joint, space underneath the knee cap, then the hip joint and then to the vertebrae. Think of your vertebrae like different size spools stacked on top of each other with round "sponges" in between that act as shock absorbers, When we think of making space between the vertebrae the sponges literally become marshmallows, light and airy, fluid goes in and you have more spine health. So now make space between the vertebrae all the way up. Relax, then do it again. Keep all Coat muscles turned off.

The way our brain helps us to stack all the time is to understand this concept of Kiss and Tell. We activate the joints by moving them and making space to tell the brain the joint is fully functional using anatomy awareness or Movement Mapping™. When you know where your joints are you focus your attention and your brain understands this is where you make space. The inside of your body doesn't look like the outside. We need to activate the Corset, the invisible part so we can stack it and set and forget it. We don't want to be supported and stiff by blowing up our outer muscles, or feel like we're hanging from an imaginary string from the sky. We are not stretched, stiff, or suspended, we are stacked from the ground up with space between the joints. By practicing Kiss and Tell, we touch, separate and make space. Every time you stand or sit, ask yourself, "Am I stacked with space?"

You're not where you think you are, you're somewhere else instead.

Your spine is an Apple Core, with a Tootsie Pop Head.

Your brain thinks in pictures, your spine is stacked with space,

Update your GPS, to burn more calories while moving place to place.

Chapter Four
Secret Four

To Lose the Pooch, No More Sit-Ups

Workout Whore

For many years I was a junkie workout whore
I did cardio, Kegels, and crunches until I discovered more
The shape is from the inside, the Corset then the Coat
If timing is off at all, you won't rid the bloat
It's been a few years without cardio and crunches
My shape is better than ever and I still enjoy my lunches!

"Hold your stomach in, squeeze, pull in, and hold it!! In fact, you're gonna have to hold it the rest of your life, honey, if you want a nice waist. That's all I heard growing up," my high school friend Maggie complained. "Now nothing works!" Maggie came to me looking for a change in her shape like most women who come to me. She wanted a smaller waist, a flat stomach, and to get rid of the belly bloat, trimming down the midsection.

The first thing we need to do is get the picture out of our mind that we need to sculpt or squeeze on the outside for a shape. The shape comes from the inside first.

First, we tighten and tone and make a real responsive well-trained Corset, then we add muscles, the outer abdominal musculature on top, the Coat, the obliques, and the rectus abdominis, which can definitely make our shape better.

But we are doing it backwards and it's increasing the pooch, pain, and peeing.

This means if you pull your navel in or do a sit-up, you have just sabotaged your Corset to the Coat sequence of activation.

You might as well go outside with no undergarments!

It isn't that doing sit-ups is bad. It's about doing them in the correct order. Unless you use your Corset first, you're just going to make lumpy, bumpy muscles.

We have turned on the Corset, now it's time to lace it for the hourglass shape.

THE CORRECT ORDER of activation IS IMPERATIVE.

During the pre-activation phase of the Corset, remember, the diaphragm pushes everything down, the pelvic floor bounces things back up, and sides narrow and compress the waist.

The back and sides of the Corset is thoracolumbar fascia, and is like the cotton on the Corset—it doesn't stretch. The laces of the Corset are on the front; they are the transverse abdominal, or TA muscles. They go horizontally from side to side. These muscles contract and release so they also need to have tone.

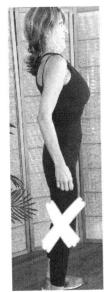

When you consciously pull in your tummy in, or do a sit up, you're using your transverse abdominis muscle, which are like the front laces on the Corset. The Corset can no longer fire in a timely sufficient manner, only late, and after the outside conscious squeeze or contraction.

The problem is, since the TA muscles are part of the inner Corset and can also be borrowed as a voluntary Coat muscle, like a sit up or when you pull in your tummy in, once this happens you've already sabotaged yourself. No longer will the pre-activation and automatic compression and narrowing of your waist happen, which is what the Corset does, because the

TA, the laces, are being borrowed by the Coat. If the Corset doesn't fire first, the TA won't have tone and you will be loose for a pooch.

We are doing things in the wrong order and won't be able to lace our Corset so we can "set it and forget it."

Remember the toothpaste tube? If you squeeze from the outside without appropriate tension with the laces of the Corset, you will have a blow out, and the pressure will need to go somewhere!

The shape comes from the inside. You cannot sculpt it from the outside. Timing is everything.

First the Corset then the Coat.

First you found your Corset by turning off your Coat and the difference between tension and relaxation. Then you rebooted the Corset with imagery and visualization with the Parasol and Reed exercise, updated your brain map with Apple Core Spine and Tootsie Pop Head.

Now we are going to continue with visualization to help you with the correct sequence from the Corset to the Coat and lace our laces so we can strengthen our Corset.

We are going to learn how to pack our suitcase before we duct tape the outside and avoid the "alien" belly, that low belly pooch that appears when you do a sit-up or cough.

Exercise

BE A BABY

Lie down, bend legs, feet underneath knee, toes slightly wider than heels, arms out on floor, heel of hands down. Use a small towel underneath the head under the largest bump on back of head NOT the neck.

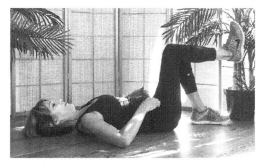

Activate the Reed Hangar as you feel the shoulder blades sink into the ground. Sunset the ribs.

Send your Sitz bones down into the ground and plug them in, making sure you're not arching your back and keep your pelvis absolutely still. First activate the Reed, then lift one bent leg up. If your belly pops out like an 'alien' belly or a pooch when you do this, your Corset is not strong enough yet and we must continue to heal it. Start slowly by hovering one foot, then work up to both legs off the ground in a bent leg position always using the Reed. Think about it, babies cried all day lying on their backs with their arms and legs flailing WITHOUT an alien belly or pooch popping up, and they did this for hours using only their inner Corset without any help from the Coat.

This can help you get the correct order from the Corset to the Coat.

Chapter Five
Secret Five

Don't work your Ass off, you'll work your Ass off of you!

Where did it go, where did it go, it used to be perky and spry

I didn't notice my booty until I had Rudy, I think it was Fourth of July

I can tell you clearly and stay on point, not let the mind wander about,

It was after his birth, my girth filled an earth that I wanted to cry and pout!

My bum is falling, my bum is falling, how oh how can it be?

Shouldn't the sky fall instead so my ass doesn't pick on me?

Cindy didn't rehab her Corset properly after she had her kids and struggled to keep the weight off, so she compensated with what she knows and feels, her voluntary Coat muscles. So she squeezes and clenches her butt to make her feel skinnier and more pulled in. Cindy got rid of the extra weight, but the habit of clenching never went away.

Even women who have not had babies or women who engage in sports and do a lot of Coat activities, squeeze their Winky by clenching their butt cheeks and inner thighs, squeezing all the time strengthening those muscles. The muscles get used to it and don't even know they're turned on all the time. So the brain says "If you're never going to let go I'm just going to scar them into place." So women get scarring in the butt muscle tissue.

It's like that pain between your shoulder blades, the thick strings that you go massage because they are held into position all the time. Muscles get tight and more scar tissue develops.

This happens with the butt muscle too, because we are not holding ourselves up the right way.

A lot of pain we experience as get older is from holding an inappropriate amount of tension in the wrong parts of our body.

We talked about how pulling your navel in all day was using only Coat muscle, sabotaging your ability to pre-activate your Corset for a smaller waist. It's the same with squeezing or clenching your butt, whether it's conscious or a habit you developed, You are working only the Coat and there IS still the timing element, from the inside to the outside.

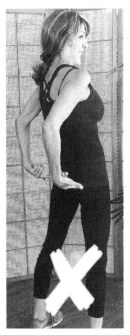

If you hold yourself tense all day, keeping your butt clenched, it will get tense and bunch up or slacken and your inner thigh muscles will get thick or balled up at the crotch, leading to shapeless legs. Who wants that, especially if it's avoidable?

The brain does whatever you tell it to do and not necessarily with the most efficient route or sequence of activation.

You're not meant to clench your butt all day. It's not what primarily holds you up, and you cannot fire your Corset properly if you do so.

Plus, your butt will disappear, like with older men who have no butts. They are the worst clenchers of all. Look for the bagginess in the butt of their pants, meaning the butts have all seized up and are now gone. Why? A habit starting around 10 years old and to be revealed in the next book.

To build a better booty, again it's the Corset that's responsible for the lift!

Remember the shape comes from the inside. There's no engaging of anything unless it's after the Corset. If the Corset fires late, it won't matter how many squats you do you.

Rigging on a Boat

Think of the floor of the core, the pelvic floor muscles are like rigging on a boat. If you pull in one side it affects the other. Or, if the rigging is not mounted correctly, if it's too loose, the sails will start slackening and folding, just like our bodies and we start leaking, if they are too tight something will rip like a torn hamstring, or even a hernia, because movement is restricted.

The rigging hoists the gluteal muscles via tendons and ligaments at the top of the leg inside the pelvis. Every time you take a step when you have your Corset on, it hoists, lifting and stretching the rigging, maintaining proper tension and function.

We all need a hoisting mechanism that works. In other words, a Corset that works, when sails slacken, it's the butt and boobs, if too tense and tight, you will be left with a derrière dent.

So there goes your booty and it isn't because of your son Rudy!

Can you see now why it's pointless to build a booty without your Corset and the rigging in place? If your rigging is faulty, don't expect to ever have a perky booty!

We have to stop clenching the butt and the Winky for this pulley system to work.

Remember it is all about timing, from the Corset to the Coat. The Corset must be triggered, so the rigging hoists the sails up the right way and hoists the booty up from the inside out. Then squat away!

During these exercises, your immediate first reaction is going to be to squeeze your butt and clench. Don't do it. Your Corset knows what to do if you let it.

Exercise

FIRESTICK

To access the hoisting mechanism, and build a better booty, slimmer thighs and ankles, we have to separate what has been frozen together, the booty and the legs, with Movement Mapping™ which is also another great exercise for bladder control!

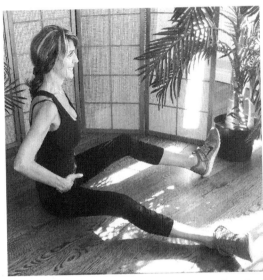

Sit on your Sitz bones, ether on a chair or the floor whatever is easiest to maintain Snowman, Hangar, Sunset and Tootsie Pop Head, it's crucial to be positioned correctly and NOT sitting on your sacrum. Keep the knees bent with the heel on the ground. Then you can activate the Reed. Now think of a caveman. He has a stick with a point on the end that he rubs on a rock with a hole in it to start a fire. This is the image you're going to have in your mind. We are going to do the same thing with our ball and socket hip joint, right where the underwear line would be and deep inside. That's where we need to focus our attention.

Imagine the leg bone goes straight up, the femur is straight, long and in one piece all the way down below the kneecap. You are going to roll it from the inside of the joint, way up high in one piece. Every time you rotate you are lifting and strengthening your pelvic floor. The pelvic floor has to expand and contract. You literally tacking down one side and then moving the other, roll in, roll out, roll in, roll out, focus deep in the joint, otherwise all the muscles around the butt and thighs completely take over the whole movement, moving your leg a lot, so focus almost like there's no movement at all. It's very deep.

BABY BRIDGE

This isn't about strengthening your thighs and your butt, it's about the Corset's hoisting mechanism, it's about pulling everything in and up before you put on the Coat.

The number one priority in this exercise is to turn off the clenching and the Winking. You have to relax your butt and your anus or butt hole. It's going to be hard to get your butt up in the air but you don't have to do it for long, do it for as long as you can get it right, then go back down and rest a second. We will be working on stamina.

Lie on your back, bent legs, feet underneath the knees, slightly turned out feet. You can put a small ball or yoga block between your knees and squeeze there a little, but not the butt.

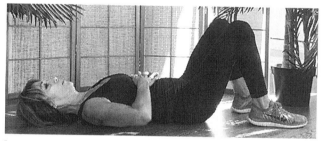 Heels plugged into floor socket. Activate Plunger Feet. Sitz bones directed down. Ribs in Sunset position, fold hands across ribs to make sure they stay down and keep them down and completely on the ground during this exercise, Hangar, Reed.

Send the Sitz bones up toward the calves to raise the pelvis off ground. You're going to want to clench. Stop and try again. The part you're lifting is below the ribs. Feel your scapula on the ground and feel your rib cage push down while sending your Sitz bones towards your calves, no clenching no Winking. Keep activating the Reed. Hold for as long as you can. Smack butt to make sure it's soft and the whole rib cage is on the ground. After everything is in position you can add the Coat muscle by doing little pulses, lifting up a little bit, feel the contraction on the outside.

Keep sending the Sitz bones towards the calves just in that direction. Get your spine very long. To come back down, it's more of a landing. Keep heels plugged in activating Toilet Plunger Feet, keep spine elongated. Use Reed and direct the Sitz bones down towards the heel sockets in the floor. The first thing that touches 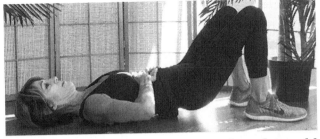 the ground are your Sitz bones into the socket. Keep the pelvis stable.

Note: The pelvis lifts and lowers all at once, there is no 'rolling up' through the vertebre, Instead, send the Sitz bones up which brings along a few vertebre, then back down to touch for the landing.

Chapter Six
Secret Sex

Why be satisfied with a fizzling sizzle,
when you can have a KABOOM!

I stopped having sex it was too laborious
It took too long to stimulate my 'clitorious'.
My sphincters were overworked and burdened from the day
They wanted to sleep and not be asked to play.

When I realized I was doing it wrong, using only my
sphincters to sing the orgasm song
The outer layer was all that I felt, and told doing Kegels
would make my man melt.
But no, it's not true, Kegels are only icing on the cake
The innermost layers needed to partake.
So I trained it with imagery, that was my new plan
He feels snug all the way up, and I have a firm grip on my man.

*S*he is sixty-two, and feels young again.

It was there all along. After years of hardship and pain, she stopped trying so hard and allowed the effortless beauty to unfold.

She stopped the acrobats and learned how to use her body, realizing what she needed all these years was already inside of her and just needed to become reacquainted with an internal truth, her Corset.

She began looking after herself to be a better woman and partner, to enhance intimacy as well as her physical sensation. She became faster and easier to please.

She realized it was never about the fuse, it was always about the gunpowder on the other side!

Laura has been reading the *7 Secrets to a Sexy Silhouette* and has reawakened her Corset. Laura is you and me.

Up until now we have trained only the Kegel muscle, the one we feel and have been working on for so long. It IS important, because that's where all the nerves are and it's highly functional with lots of sensation, but it tricks your brain into thinking that there's a lot going on down there.

It's not that Kegels aren't important, it's just that they are not enough.

Kegels are the fuse for the dynamite on the other side, and we DO need a fuse.

So you have a choice.

You can just work on the fuse, it's not so bad, it can give you that little sizzle, or little blurb of an orgasm that sometimes barely keeps the flame lit. It just goes out and is not very satisfying but it's what you feel. It's just a fuse.

But if you want the Big Bang, you have to lace your Corset by focusing on the Reed.

All of the pelvic floor layers work together from the inside to outside, increasing the squeeze from the engorgement of ALL layers when you have an orgasm, so it's more intense. The pelvic floor layers need to be able to swell up and squeeze out for it to have the contractions and rhythmic waves. That's where the stimulation comes from, pelvic congestion and release.

Things start happening in the body from the innermost strongest trampoline layer, which has been awakened. The brain can now allocate new resources with the Reed exercise, such as new nerve endings, increased blood flow, and removal of toxic waste. You are literally building the gunpowder reserve and keeping your guns oiled. No more dryness!

If the outer Kegel muscles are tight or tense, there is no way to build gunpowder and keep the guns oiled. It's just like the faucet and the water main pipe in Secret Two, we have to turn it off to go up through.

So Kegels for sex is exhausting and unnecessary because now we have the Reed, which is much better as it engorges all three layers with a load of combustion right behind it.

The Reed improves your body's function by enhancing your capacity for more gunpowder, resulting in a much larger bang, The Big One!

You don't need lubricants, you just need to keep your gun oiled and he will feel the difference all the way up the three floors instead of just feeling a tight outside Kegel (Coat) that he pokes through only to discover a vastness of outer space on the other side, barely able to hold onto him.

Fantasy and Imagery for a Snuggly Man Cave

If you already experience the fantasy which is one of the things that helps you have a more intense sexual response, you can now take the fantasy and direct it inward, using it to have your body physiologically prepared to respond to give you what Dr. Theresa calls the Big Bang!

Fantasy can ONLY take you so far. Fantasy with imagery will overlap. Your fantasies are outside of your body; the imagery is going to be helpful to use inside your body.

Imagery actually hooks into helping your brain improve your body.

By doing things in the correct order, which means understanding how your Corset works with the Coat, you get better muscle response and increased engorgement of the pelvic floor layers for the Big Bang orgasm!

That means a lot more fun with a lot less work! KABOOM!!!

It's about functioning and keeping that part of you alive and vibrant. If that part is alive and vibrant, you are alive and vibrant.

Getting older should make your sex life better, not worse. We don't have to depreciate. Put yourself as a priority.

Pooch, pain, peeing, and sexual dysfunction are NOT what's to be expected and you're not withering away. Just protect and continue to build up your supplies.

Even if you don't have sex, you still want to be sexy, don't you?

As we get older, our hormones change, so these exercises simply put the juice back in our sex life.

It's not about performing; it's about this experience that you have your whole life, knowing how to pull your body together. This means knowing your body, but many of us are in our 50s and don't know our body at all. We want vitality and sexuality, and that means addressing all of our parts at every age and stage of life.

By the way, if you stop having sex because you accidentally leak urine, you will find that these exercises not only help you with sexual response, but if you happen to have a leaking problem, it's really going to help that too!

Exercise

Besides the Reed exercise, I love Wag the Tail as pulls on the tight pelvic floor layers, in order to engorge all of them equally.

WAG THE TAIL

On your hands and knees, hands underneath boobs with fingers turned slightly inward. Hangar, Sunset ribs, and a fully elongated spine position with Apple Core, Tootsie Pop Head and aligned with Snowman. You may need to put a rolled towel under your ankles to help you maintain Toilet Plunger Feet with toes slightly wider than heels. Imagine you can uncurl your tightly tucked tailbone up to the

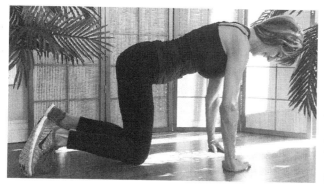

sky and wag it as fast as you can 20 times without moving your butt or with any other visible movement. Stop and repeat. Your body remains absolutely still.

This will help build your gunpowder supply, have a longer fuse and Big Bang without exhausting yourself in the process. Make sure you wag your tail fast and hard without moving your butt or anything else and without pinching off your Winky. Keep the speed of contraction up. It improves sexual functioning, keeps things toned and lively, and helps you control the 'flow' when you pee.

Chapter Seven
Secret Seven

Don't Die by a Desk Sentence

Sit at your desk, sit by the sea,

Sit Well wherever, which sits well with me!

Sit on a stump, pick up your key, bend over, do laundry, get down on one knee,

Stay mindful, mind your movement, and thy mood with thee,

Stay on track my friends, and watch life change exponentially!

I teach an inner core class at Torrance Memorial Hospital for the community. On occasion, I am interviewed for the hospital's magazine, called *The Pulse,* or asked to speak at local businesses.

A few weeks ago, the physical therapist who was scheduled to speak at the home office of Pentel Corp. for the executives during lunch wasn't available, so they asked if I was interested in subbing. "Sure," I said. My contact loved the title and assured me they couldn't wait for the presentation "How to Avoid the Desk Sentence™".

During lunch, the first question I asked was, "How many of you feel pain between the shoulder blades, neck, low back from sitting at your desk all day?" Out of 15 lunchtime executives, 10 raised their hands. The presentation was halfway over and I noticed a few people changing postures. Others even noticed that one of the executives looked thinner and taller. They commented to him. He had no idea that his posture was any different, especially since he was eating lunch. His grin became as wide as can be!

After I showed them how to avoid the "desk sentence" by what I am going to teach you, something wonderful but very common happened. After the hour, when I asked again how many people have less pain now than when they walked in an hour ago, eight people happily raised their hands, smiling with happy wide eyes. Their backs and shoulders didn't hurt anymore!

The next day, the Torrance Memorial Hospital's coordinator received an email from Pentel Corp. thanking them for the presentation, indicating that, "This was the most informative and thought-provoking presentation that the staff has encountered." and "We would like Kathleen to come back in the near future."

This is what I am talking about. Stay with this journey. The changes can be either subtle or drastic, but always faster than you can imagine when you do Imagine. It's the nervous system, which is way faster!

This is what I shared with Pentel Corp.

How to Avoid the Desk Sentence

A lot of people sit at their desk with what we call space bar thumbs. They take their eyes and their thumbs and they move into the computer. It's stressful; you're not burning any calories and it makes your boobs all droopy.

You don't want to be stiff, you want to be stacked.

We are going to set our arms up with the energy going down from the shoulder to the elbow and out the ring finger, not the thumb, to have more comfort at work and less pain between your shoulder blades.

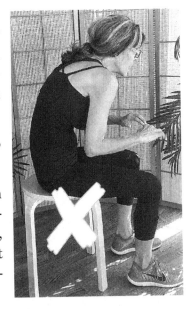

Sit at your desk on your Sitz bones, Toilet Plunger Feet underneath the knees, stacked like a Snowman in alignment with space. Tootsie

Pop Head and set your eyes back inside your skull.

Ribs maintain a soft downward exhalation position, Sunset, Hangar, and allow your elbows to drop at the side. Activate the Reed.

The strongest alignment of the spine goes through your ring finger. When you lift your arms up, you're going to lift them up by the ring

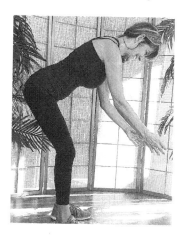

finger instead of the thumb. First, let your elbows hang like there's a little weight on them and lift your ring finger up first.

To maintain alignment pretend you're typing like an old-fashioned secretary from the 60s without a keyboard, to get the feeling of your ring finger pumping up and down, keep your elbows hanging.

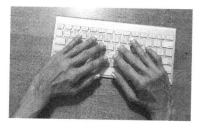

When you type, your thumbs are positioned on the space bar and your typing is coming from the ring finger. Feel your hands stay light on the keyboard.

How to activate your Corset to perk up your booty while picking up your Grandbaby or puppy.

Activate Toilet Plunger feet and the Reed. Maintain Apple Core,

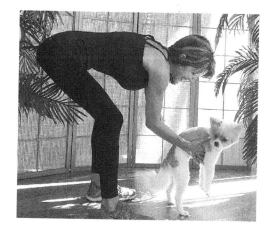

Tootsie Pop Head, Snowman, Stacked with Space. Sunset and Hangar. Inhale air goes into Bikini, karate chop at the underwear line, send your Sitz bones back, along with your tailbone and reach for baby or puppy, exhale and lift with ease. Spine stays long throughout the movement.

Last but not least...Sleep well!

New research shows that now we understand how to flush unnecessary debris out of our brains, the stuff that accumulates by all of the hard work your brain is doing. It literally is a flush of brain fluid. It washes out all the cognitive crap or clutter that you have stored in there. If you don't sleep, it just keeps building up.

To clean up the home office, the brain, so to speak, where all information and incoming data comes in and is stored, we must SLEEP.

Review this book often and practice the exercises as much as you can think about them. Commit to your health, practice patience, and gratefulness daily. You already know the research on practicing thankfulness and gratitude. It does wonders to decrease stress (belly fat) and renews your passions. La Dolce Vita

For beautiful eyes, look for the good in others

For beautiful lips, speak only words of kindness

For poise, walk in the knowledge you are never alone.

Audrey Hepburn

About the Author

Kathleen Pagnini, Aged 57

Inner Core and Pelvic Floor Specialist

Prior to studying the 'inner' core Kathleen has spent over 35 years focusing on the 'outer' core as an International Fitness and Pilates Expert. She has also won Aerobic Championships and Bodybuilding Contests.

Originally from Los Angeles, she has lived all over the world and has owned and managed multiple fitness facilities. She recently relocated to Redondo Beach, California.

In 2009, after creating the "Pilates and Chocolate" DVD that sells on Amazon, Kathleen was selected to mentor privately with world renowned, Dr. Theresa Nesbitt, OBGYN, Women's Wellness Specialist, to study and develop a Revolutionary Scientific Breakthrough System for women's health; addressing leaking urine issues, back pain, better sex, and how to have a smaller waist... without maniac workouts, without pills, pads, surgery, Kegels or crunches.

It's a 'work in' program, a relaxation program.

Today Kathleen joins a handpicked team of experts worldwide led by Dr. Theresa, as she embarks on this new frontier for women's health.

Kathleen is the host of the show "No Pause Menopause" on WBTVN.TV Women's TV Network every Monday.

She is the creator of *The Corset And The Coat* online eCourse and author of the book, *7 Secrets to a Sexy Silhouette*.

Made in the USA
San Bernardino, CA
05 April 2018